# Table of Contents

# INTRODUCTION

The paleo diet is the ultimate throwback diet: It promotes a return to eating as our ancestors did in the Stone Age. "This regimen is based on the idea that our bodies do best when fueled by foods that existed in the Paleolithic era, before agriculture came along 10,000 or so years ago. That means no sugar, grain, dairy, legumes, or beans on the paleo diet. No highly processed cookies or cakes. And no foods with added hormones or artificial ingredients. As for what's on the paleo menu, think meat, fish, vegetables, and limited amounts of fruit, nuts, and seeds. "That's about it," Dr. Hyman says. It may not seem like much, but what you're left with are nutrient-packed foods, many of which are excellent sources of fiber, which helps you feel satisfied and full. Should you embrace the caveman way? Here's what to know — including benefits and risks to be aware of, whom the diet is good for, and who should consult a physician before jumping on the bandwagon. This way of eating may sound extreme — you're cutting out entire food groups, after all — but it can be a healthy alternative to the typical American diet, which is high in grain-based, sugary foods loaded with highly processed fats and oils "Eliminating carbohydrates and processed foods may not be a bad idea — especially in the case of processed carbs — and may result in weight loss, since the bulk of the American diet comes from carbs," says Adrienne Youdim, MD, an associate clinical professor of medicine at the University of California at Los Angeles David Geffen School of Medicine.

# PALEO DIET: WHAT YOU CAN (AND CAN'T) EAT

When you cut out processed foods and their empty calories — things like cookies, potato chips, butter, sweets, and sugary drinks — you'll lose weight (as long as you have weight to lose). But the benefits may extend beyond your waistline. One review suggests that, when compared with other diets, the paleo approach led to small improvements in blood pressure in people with signs of metabolic syndrome, fasting blood sugar, and triglycerides, which are fats found in the blood that can increase your risk of stroke, heart attack, and death.

## What Are the Risks Associated With the Paleo Diet?

While cutting out whole food groups can certainly help your weight loss efforts (take, for example, the popularity of the all-meat carnivore diet, which most dietitians don't recommend), you may run the risk of missing out on key nutrients. For instance, some experts caution against the paleo diet because eliminating dairy can leave you with lower levels of calcium and vitamin D. Over time, this could put you at risk of developing osteoporosis, bone fractures, or rickets. (3)

Many also worry because the diet is often interpreted as meat-centric. "Some use the paleo philosophy as an excuse to eat too much meat and too few plant-based foods," Hyman says. If you're not careful about the types of protein you eat, the diet can put you at increased risk of developing cardiovascular disease, Dr. Youdim says. Red meat, for instance, is high in saturated fats, which can raise blood cholesterol levels and increase the risk of heart disease.

## Who Might Benefit From Trying the Paleo Diet?

People who've had trouble following diets that require them to count calories or macronutrients may find this way of eating helpful. With the paleo diet, there are foods you can eat and foods you can't eat, plain and simple. That doesn't mean sticking to the diet is easy — in fact, many find it tough to follow, Youdim says — but it requires diligent food prep rather than calculating and journaling. Hyman says there's emerging research that the paleo diet (or the ketogenic diet, which is a more aggressive low-carb, high-fat diet) may help manage type 2 diabetes. One study found that people with type 2 diabetes who followed a paleo diet for two weeks saw improvements to their blood sugar, lipid profiles, and insulin sensitivity compared with those who stuck to a more conventional diet filled with salt, dairy, whole grains, and legumes. Another study found that within 12 weeks, a paleo diet helped people with type 2 diabetes reduce their body fat, increase insulin sensitivity, and improve blood sugar control, among other benefits. In the same randomized controlled trial, those participants who did paleo and exercised also improved their heart health and boosted their lean muscle mass. (6) People with type 2 diabetes are two times as likely to die of heart disease as those people without the condition. Nevertheless, it's important to note that both of these studies were small, with only 24 and 32 participants, respectively, so more research will be needed to confirm the results.

*Should Certain People Avoid the Paleo Diet?*

Even though some research suggests the paleo diet can help people with type 2 diabetes, they should consult a doctor first. Any drastic reduction in carb intake is worrisome for this group, especially for those who are on insulin; your blood sugar levels may plummet if you don't make changes to your medications first. Furthermore, while you might find claims online about the paleo diet helping treat autoimmune conditions, more research is needed before knowing what role, if any, this diet may play a role in treating ailments such as multiple sclerosis (MS), inflammatory bowel disease (IBD), and celiac disease.

# HEART DISEASE AND PALEO

Obesity, heart disease, and diabetes: These are just a few of the health conditions that proponents of the Paleolithic diet, or caveman diet, blame on our sedentary lifestyles and modern way of eating, which is loaded with sugar, fat, and processed foods. Their proposed solution? Cut modern foods from our diet and return to the way our early hunter-gatherer ancestors ate. To get an idea of what that means, we turned to the experts, including Loren Cordain, PhD, a professor emeritus at Colorado State University in Fort Collins and the author of The Paleo Diet; Erin Holley, RD, of The Ohio State University Wexner Medical Center in Columbus; and Lona Sandon, PhD, RD, an associate professor of clinical nutrition at the University of Texas Southwestern Medical Center in Dallas.

For starters, to be and stay healthy on the paleo diet, Dr. Cordain says that you'll need to exercise regularly while following a strict diet made up of only foods that can be hunted and gathered. In its purest form, the paleo diet allows you to eat just those foods that humans ate when they first roamed the planet about 2.5 million years ago. The diet can improve your health by eliminating high-fat and processed foods that have little nutritional value and too many calories. This plan emphasizes loading up on fruits and vegetables that are bursting with healthy vitamins, minerals, and fiber, which fills you up faster so you eat less, helping curb weight gain, according to research.

You'll lose weight because anytime you restrict entire food groups, your calorie intake tends to be lower, Dr. Sandon says. And according to the National Heart, Lung, and Blood Institute, whenever you burn more calories than you consume, you'll lose weight. The focus on lean protein, fruits, and vegetables over calorie- and sodium-rich processed foods can also contribute to weight loss, according to research on other diet plans that incorporate these tenets of healthy eating. But Sandon points out that the paleo diet wasn't created to be a weight loss diet. Although nuts and seeds are allowed on this diet, they can be high in calories, and people who want to lose weight will have to limit their nut consumption.

What Does Research Say About the Paleo Diet?

So what does the science say about the paleo diet? Some research suggests that the health claims hold water. A review that analyzed four randomized, controlled trials totaling 159 participants found that the paleo diet led to more short-term improvements in some risk factors for chronic disease (including waist circumference and fasting blood sugar) compared with diets used as controls. In fact, many scientists have expressed concern that we do not yet have enough evidence to make any strong claims about the paleo diet's health benefits, especially its long-term effects. In response to the first review.

Among their arguments: Some of the results were not statistically significant, nor did they show "any important clinical effects." They concluded that they did not believe that the results of the review showed any evidence in favor of the paleo diet, and they called for more care in reaching health recommendations for the general public.

## Foods to Eat and Avoid on the Paleo Diet

On the paleo diet, you'll find fewer processed foods, but you'll also need to cut out all grains, legumes, and most dairy. Here's a closer look at the eating plan.

What to Eat

Although the paleo diet isn't proven to work, if you want to give this eating plan a try, you'll need to prioritize fueling up on lots of natural foods and natural fats, including these options:

Lean cuts of beef, pork, and poultry, preferably grass-fed, organic, or free-range selections

Game animals, such as quail, venison, and bison

Eggs, but no more than six a week and preferably free-range

Fish, including shellfish

Fruit, such as strawberries, cantaloupe, mango, and figs

Nonstarchy vegetables, such as asparagus, onions, and peppers

Nuts and seeds, including almonds, cashews, walnuts, and pumpkin seeds

Olive oil, flaxseed oil, and walnut oil, in moderation

What to Avoid

Similarly, any foods that were not easily available to Paleolithic humans are off-limits in this diet, Holley explains. That means processed foods — many of which contain added butter, margarine, and sugar — should not be a part of the paleo diet. The same goes for dairy, which may not have been accessible to Paleolithic humans, and legumes, which many proponents of the diet believe are not easily digestible by the body. Keep in mind that some versions of the paleo diet are less strict than others and allow some dairy products or legumes, like peanuts, Holley says. Foods to avoid:

All dairy products, including milk, cheese, yogurt, and butter

Cereal grains, such as wheat, rye, rice, and barley

Legumes, like beans, peanuts, and peas

Starchy vegetables, such as potatoes (and some even say sweet potatoes)

Sweets, including all forms of candy as well as honey and sugar

Artificial sweeteners

Sugary soft drinks and fruit juices

Processed and cured meats, such as bacon, deli meats, and hot dogs

*Highly processed foodsA Sample Menu of What to Eat on the Paleo Diet*

The paleo diet has become one of the most popular eating approaches out there, so you won't have trouble finding a bounty of paleo-friendly recipes online and on bookshelves. But if you're a beginner, consider this one-day sample menu of the paleo diet to get you started.

Breakfast Onion and spinach omelet with liver pâté

Lunch Tuna wrapped in lettuce with almonds

Snack Hard-boiled eggs

Dinner Beef bourguignon

Dessert Ice cream made from coconut milk

Possible Risks and Benefits of Trying the Paleo Diet

While the paleo diet is certainly not a cure-all, it does come with some potential benefits. But that doesn't mean it's for everyone — there are also some risks you should be aware of before diving in.

Potential Pros of Following the Paleo Diet: It's Nutritious and Easy to Follow, and It Involves Exercise

There are a handful of benefits you'll potentially reap from following the paleo diet.

First, by eating fruits and vegetables, you'll get many of the essential vitamins and minerals you need.

Also, the diet is simple. You eat the foods that are acceptable and avoid those that are not — there's no meal plan or diet cycle to stick to.

## IS THE PALEO DIET GOOD FOR HEART HEALTH?

As with type 2 diabetes, the paleo diet may or may not be good for your heart. It comes down to how you follow the eating approach. If you were to eat an unlimited amount of red meat (which the paleo diet technically allows), you would most likely see your heart health suffer. While experts applaud the omission of packaged and processed foods like cakes, cookies, chips, and candy — which are well known to be bad for your ticker — they're not crazy about the fact that paleo doesn't allow you to eat whole grains, legumes, and most dairy. Whole grains in particular have been linked with better cholesterol levels, as well as a reduced risk of stroke, obesity, and type 2 diabetes, according to the American Heart Association. These are all comorbidities of heart disease, per the National Institute of Diabetes and Digestive and Kidney Diseases. The gist? Talk to your doctor before trying the paleo diet for heart disease. They will be able to tell you if it's a good fit and, if so, how you should approach the plan for optimal health.

Can the Paleo Diet Help You Manage Autoimmune Diseases?

Although research on the paleo diet's possible role in helping manage autoimmune diseases is limited at best, researchers' and paleo proponents' interest in this prospect isn't waning. There's even a niche paleo diet for this very purpose called the autoimmune paleo diet.nWhile proponents of the paleo diet say they've anecdotally seen the diet help control inflammatory bowel disease, psoriasis, eczema, multiple sclerosis, celiac disease, and Hashimoto's thyroiditis, research on these effects is lacking. Definitely don't expect paleo to be a panacea for any autoimmune disease you may be managing, and be sure to consult your doctor before diving in.

You could lose weight following a Paleolithic diet — and quickly, too, depending on how strictly you adhere to eating the foods from the allowed list and how much physical exercise you add to your daily routine. In the long term, you have to be sure that you're getting calcium and other nutrients you're missing by not having dairy products and certain grains. Some paleo-approved foods, such as salmon and spinach, contain calcium, so you have to be sure you're including them in your diet. It would be a good idea to check with a registered dietitian, too, to make sure you're meeting your calcium and other nutrient needs.

On the whole, the paleo diet is not a bad choice, Holley says. If someone follows the diet by cutting out processed food, processed meats, and sugar-sweetened beverages and swaps them for more fruits, vegetables, and healthy fats, they're likely to see some health benefits.

"One thing to consider is how extreme you want to take it," says Holley, noting that some versions of the diet are more restrictive than others, limiting foods like dairy or peanut butter. It could be overwhelming to cut out a bunch of food groups all at once. Holley suggests trying small incremental changes instead. Overall, the diet is not for everyone, but it could be helpful to some, Holley says. "It's important for each person to carefully understand the diet before they jump in." Before making any changes to your diet or exercise plan, be sure to speak with your physician to make sure that the changes you would like to make align with your personal health needs.

## What is The Paleo Diet?

Prior to starting a new diet plan, consult with your healthcare provider or a registered dietitian, especially if you have an underlying health condition. Get ready to channel your inner hunter-gatherer if you're preparing to follow the paleo diet. This diet only allows foods readily available before the dawn of agriculture. Some of the foods you've enjoyed in the past may now be off-limits, as the diet eliminates food groups like grains and dairy. With careful planning and preparation, though, you can enjoy various nutritious meals on the paleo diet.

*What You Can Eat*
There's no one "official" set of paleo diet guidelines. Most proponents have taken what they believe to be true about ancestral eating and developed recommendations based on this.1 However, there are several divergences of opinion that you may see within each subgroup of compliant and non-compliant foods.

Meat and Fish

Some paleo proponents also recommend paying attention to the way the animals were raised. The strictest guidelines advise only eating grass-fed beef, free-range poultry, and wild-caught fish.

Beef

Poultry

Pork

Seafood

Fish

Veal

Venison

Eggs

Eggs are a staple in the paleo diet, and make a great option for quick breakfasts or snacks. Some strict guidelines recommend eating only free-range, organic eggs – while less rigid ones suggest any eggs are fine.


Vegetables

Non-starchy vegetables are a vital component of this diet, and for a good reason – they're packed with vitamins, minerals, and phytochemicals. Paleo proponents diverge a bit on starchy vegetables. Most paleo plans allow certain starchy vegetables like sweet potatoes but place white potatoes off-limits. Some followers refuse to include any tubers, while others have decided to embrace all starchy vegetables, including white potatoes.

Leafy greens (spinach, kale, chard)

Asparagus

Mushrooms

Zucchini

Bell peppers

Hot peppers

Cabbage


Fruits

You'll be able to enjoy your favorite fruits on the paleo diet. Some paleo plans limit higher-sugar fruits (like grapes or pineapple) if you're trying to lose weight, while others don't place any restrictions on these naturally sweet treats.

Berries

Cherries

Apples

Citrus

Nuts and Seeds

You're free to graze on any other nuts and seeds except for peanuts. These are rich in good fats, making them a satiating snack to eat during the day. You also may find these in beverage form, such as unsweetened almond milk, often used as a dairy substitute for those on this diet.

Nut milks (almond, cashew)

Nut and seed butters (almond, pumpkin seed, sunflower seed)

Whole nuts and seeds

Nut and seed flours (flax meal, almond meal)

Certain Oils

There's no "official" definition of the paleo diet; different authors or researchers have alternative guidelines for recommended oils. In general, these include:

Olive oil

Coconut oil

Avocado oil

Macadamia nut oil

Walnut oil

*What You Cannot Eat*
There are several foods eliminated from the Paleo diet. Although there is no scientific evidence backing the claims that these foods were not part of some Paleolithic people's diets, the basis for excluding them is the belief that they were not traditionally consumed.

Grains

All grains are eliminated on a paleo diet. Proponents of the diet claim that "anti-nutrients" like phytates, lectins, and gluten are bad for your body. Scientific evidence has not proven these theories to be accurate, though. For example, no current scientific evidence supports eliminating gluten unless you have celiac disease or food sensitivity to gluten.

Wheat

Oats

Quinoa

Amaranth

Cornmeal

Rice

Legumes

Legumes are a category of plants with a pod that carries seeds.4 Like grains, paleo proponents recommend avoiding all legumes due to claims regarding their high lectin and phytate content. If you do decide to follow the paleo diet, remember that this category also includes spreads like peanut butter (peanuts) and hummus (beans), as well as sauces like soy sauce and teriyaki sauce (soy).

Beans

Peas

Peanuts

Lentils

Soy

Dairy Products

The most rigid paleo guidelines exclude all dairy. These products are traditionally eliminated for two reasons: misguided belief that early humans did not eat dairy products before domestication, and some paleo proponents voiced concerns over lactose intolerance and milk protein sensitivities. Since the initial paleo push, some people have embraced certain dairy products, such as full-fat, grass-fed clarified butter, or fermented dairy like kefir.

Because there is no "official" definition for a paleo diet, it's a personal decision to include limited dairy on this diet. There is currently no solid evidence for avoiding dairy from a research-based standpoint unless you have an allergy or sensitivity.

Milk

Cheese

Butter

Yogurt

Ice cream

Throughout human history, tolerance to lactose evolved to enable many to consume dairy without any health concerns.5 There is no scientific reason to avoid dairy altogether unless you have an allergy. Even lactose-intolerant individuals can find lactose-free dairy products if desired.

Refined Sugar

You'll probably need to clear out some items from your pantry, as no refined sugar is allowed. This includes sugar that you might add to a baked good or any number of the added sugars found in ingredient lists for packaged foods. Some paleo diet plans allow small amounts of honey or maple syrup, though, so you can still occasionally create some tasty desserts.

Artificial Sweeteners

Artificial sweeteners are commonly used to add a sweet taste to foods without calories. You'll want to eliminate all artificial sweeteners on the paleo diet, as they were not around back in prehistoric times. This includes:

Sucralose

Aspartame

Acesulfame potassium

Saccharin

Certain Oils

Most paleo proponents recommend excluding the following oils from the diet:

Canola oil

Corn oil

Grapeseed oil

Peanut oil

Safflower oil

Sunflower seed oil

Soybean oil (frequently called "vegetable oil" on product labels)

These are excluded either due to a high omega-6 fatty acid content or because they are frequently GMO products.


Processed foods


If you're used to grabbing snacks or frozen meals at the grocery store, you'll need to re-evaluate those choices on a paleo diet. Our great ancestors didn't have processed snack foods to pop while binge-watching television or a microwavable TV dinner to heat up when they didn't want to cook. As such, most processed foods are off-limits on this diet.1

Recommended Timing

There's no official meal timing for the paleo diet. As long as you are choosing compliant foods, you can stick with a conventional eating schedule of three meals a day with any necessary snacks in between. Ceertain paleo proponents – like Loren Cordain, for example – do recommend abstaining from late night eating to keep in line with circadian rhythm.

There is also a growing segment of people promoting an intermittent fasting diet (specifically, the time-restricted feeding model) in conjunction with the paleo diet. In this case, you would fast for part of the day and then only eat paleo meals during an 8-hour eating window (for example, from 8am-4pm or 10am-6pm). Though research has shown some initial promising effects of intermittent fasting on weight loss measures, there is little long-term data available at this time.

Resources and Tips

While many would consider the paleo diet restrictive due to the exclusion of multiple food groups, there are still plenty of delicious and nutritious meals you can make.1 Here are a few tips to help you on your paleo journey:

Remember that meat/fish and vegetables can be the starting point for just about any meal. Experiment with the types of meat you buy, trying different cuts of beef or different types of seafood. Similarly, explore the produce section at your grocery store or hit up your local farmer's market for new types of produce. Being an adventurous shopper like this will help you continuously add variety to your meals.

Shop the sales - and shop around! If you're following strict paleo guidelines to only purchase grass-fed beef and wild-caught fish, it can start to take a toll on your wallet. Try to keep an eye out for what's on sale each week at your grocery store, and stock up when you catch a good price. Be sure to also explore the pricing from local fishmongers and butchers, local farms, or meat and fish CSA programs.6

Get creative with occasional sweet treats. While store-bought snacks and desserts are generally off-limits, you can work within the confines of the paleo diet to create your own occasional sweet treats. Regular flour can be substituted for alternatives like almond flour; sugar can be subbed out for date paste or a smidge of maple syrup or honey. You'll find tons of inspiration online for paleo-friendly desserts. Just remember that these should still be eaten only in moderation; eating them frequently is not in line with the diet's goals.

If you need some culinary inspiration, be sure to check out one of the many Paleo cookbooks on the market. You can use these cookbooks or online recipes to prepare your meal plans each week and then shop for groceries based on those ideas. That way, your kitchen is always stocked with exactly what you need.

*Modifications*
Because the paleo diet excludes several food groups, it can be difficult for some groups to meet their nutritional needs

without extra planning. If you fit one of the groups below, consider making some modifications to this diet:

Pregnant Women

There are several pluses to the paleo diet when it comes to pregnancy – in particular, an emphasis on lots of nutrient-rich produce, the inclusion of omega-3 fatty acids from fish, and limiting less-healthy processed foods. However, eliminating grains, legumes, and dairy can make it very challenging to meet energy needs, especially if a woman is struggling with food aversions to meat or fish. In addition, key prenatal nutrients like calcium and Vitamin D – frequently in dairy products – may be more challenging to meet with the exclusion of dairy.

During pregnancy, focus on what works best for your body and always check with a doctor to see if a certain diet is appropriate. If you're finding it hard to meet your needs on the paleo diet, add in one or more of the excluded food groups.

Children

Most experts agree that it's unwise to put children on a very restrictive meal plan, barring a medically-necessary diet. Forcing a child to only eat paleo-approved foods might put them at potential risk for nutritional deficiencies (for example, a lack of calcium due to the elimination of dairy) without proper planning. BPerhaps even more concerning though is that restriction in childhood can create an unhealthy relationship with food later in life. Try to maintain a neutral approach that no one food is "bad" or "good."

Endurance Athletes

For most competitive endurance athletes (barring those who practice a keto diet), getting enough carbohydrate is essential to performance. Though the paleo diet includes some carbohydrates from fruits and vegetables, the elimination of grains can leave athletes falling short.nIf you want to stick with a paleo style diet as an athlete, be sure to include plenty of starchy vegetables.8 Though some strict paleo advocates recommend avoiding these, you'll need that energy if you decide not to add grains back in.

Depending on your training and body, you may find it best to add grains back to the diet though during peak season.

Can the Paleo Diet Help Fight Autoimmune Diseases?

Critics have dismissed the paleolithic, or "caveman," diet as a fad, while its proponents have embraced the eating approach as a necessary return to the healthy simplicity of our ancient ancestors' diets. But what's the truth? And can this popular diet really help fight the inflammation that coexists with many autoimmune diseases? First, know that paleo is an anti-inflammatory diet that aims to remove sugar, legumes, most dairy, grains, and refined vegetable oils like corn and soy oil. Essentially, paleo sets out to eliminate processed, so-called modern foods from our diets. Indeed, the paleo diet gets its name from its focus on the foods ancient hunter-gatherers relied on.

Can the Paleo Diet Help Relieve Symptoms of Autoimmune Disease?

Some studies suggest that paleo really does offer benefits, like weight loss and more energy, while others show anecdotal evidence that eliminating inflammatory foods in the standard American diet — such as soda, chips, and cookies — as well as grains, legumes, and most dairy, can help people manage diseases like Crohn's disease, ulcerative colitis, rheumatoid arthritis, psoriasis, and multiple sclerosis (MS). Sounds great, right? Not so fast. Turns out, more research is needed before we can know for sure what effect this restrictive diet may have on autoimmune diseases, says Kelly Kennedy, RD, CDE, the staff dietitian at Everyday Health.

"Unfortunately, there just isn't enough scientific evidence to clearly show that following a paleo diet would be helpful for improving symptoms of an autoimmune condition," Kennedy says. "For some people, following the diet might help, but for others, it may not."

# WHAT ABOUT THE AUTOIMMUNE PALEO DIET (AIP)?

## DOES IT WORK?

If you've researched diets for autoimmune diseases online, you've likely come across the autoimmune paleo diet (AIP), which proposes to directly address gut inflammation that leads to autoimmune disease. This diet is sometimes called the autoimmune protocol diet, and depending on where you're looking, they may be one and the same, or the paleo diet may be a type of an autoimmune protocol diet. In any case, AIP is specifically geared toward reducing inflammation in the body that leads to flares for conditions like inflammatory bowel disease (IBD). (2) It focuses mainly on vegetables and meats, and tackles what some people in the holistic health community have dubbed "leaky gut," which is believed to contribute to the chronic inflammation associated with autoimmune diseases.

## How the Paleo Diet May Help Treat 5 Autoimmune Conditions

Still, some research supports the idea of using paleo to treat autoimmune conditions. Here's what you should know about paleo and its potential benefits for five well-known autoimmune conditions.

1. IBD

An estimated 3.1 million people have IBD in the United States. (3) One study found that an AIP diet can "improve clinical responses in (IBD)." The researchers monitored 18 adults with IBD who went through a six-week elimination diet followed by a five-week "maintenance phase." At the end of the study, an endoscopy was performed on the people participating. While the study found significant improvement in some people's symptoms after they went on the diet, two of the participants who had ileal strictures — a common complication of Crohn's disease — before the study began experienced worsening symptoms.

## 2. Skin Conditions Like Psoriasis and Eczema

Some paleo proponents cite the diet's ability to curb inflammation as playing a big role in improving chronic skin conditions like psoriasis and eczema. Again, more research is needed," she stresses, reiterating that a standard elimination diet is still the most recommended approach for helping with skin conditions such as eczema or psoriasis. In a 2017 survey of psoriasis patients, nearly 70 percent reported a favorable response to the paleo diet.

## 3. Multiple Sclerosis (MS)

Some current research suggests that paleo may help with MS. (5) The research — which looked at a small, uncontrolled pool of 13 people — suggests that people who adhered to the paleo diet, along with an exercise program and meditation, showed "significant improvement in fatigue." But it's unclear exactly which part of the treatment (exercise, diet, or meditation) actually helped people with their symptoms.

Healthy Eating Habits for Multiple Sclerosis

For this research, 10 out of 13 participants enrolled in a two-week study, then went on to be observed over a 12-month period. Eventually, eight people completed the study and six of them fully stuck with the paleo diet. The results were promising and suggested the need for more research down the line. "While there are anecdotal success stories, the benefit remains to be proven in a scientific study," Kennedy says.

## 4. Celiac Disease

The paleo diet includes only gluten-free foods, so it's no surprise the plan is popular among people managing celiac disease, which is marked by gluten intolerance. But the paleo diet isn't necessarily the best — and certainly isn't the only — diet option if you're managing celiac, Kennedy notes. "For [those] diagnosed with celiac disease, the results are clear: Following a gluten-free diet is necessary to control symptoms. However, any other paleo diet limitations beyond this would not affect the disease symptoms," Kennedy says.

5. Hashimoto's Thyroiditis

Hashimoto's thyroiditis is an autoimmune disease that affects the thyroid gland, and symptoms can include weight gain, depression, and fatigue. Some people point to this being a condition that can be fought off with paleo. Why? A study suggests that a low-carbohydrate diet — which effectively is partially a paleo diet — may decrease thyroid antibodies that signify Hashimoto's. (6) An additional study also showed AIP may decrease systemic inflammation and modulate the immune system. But as with all of these conditions, more research on paleo's impact needs to be conducted. If you have this condition, Kennedy urges you not to rush into paleo, arguing that there is not enough evidence out there to suggest it's effective for treating your symptoms. She notes that it is important to consult your physician for proper Hashimoto's treatment.

## Paleo Diet Short- and Long-Term Effects

The paleo diet has been one of the trendiest weight loss plans out there today, but it's rooted in our ancestors' eating habits from tens of thousands of years ago. The diet rejects many of the food groups that make up the typical American diet — including grains, dairy, sugar, and legumes. Swapping a spaghetti-and-meatballs dinner for a plate that's loaded with veggies and a lean piece of protein may not be easy, but it could be beneficial to your health.

What to Expect in the Short Term if You Try the Paleo Diet

If you're considering the paleo diet, the first challenge you'll likely encounter will be overcoming waning energy levels. (Have a tendency to get hangry? Consider yourself warned.) Without energy-rich carbs, you may feel excessively tired and in a bad mood, says Adrienne Youdim, MD, an associate clinical professor of medicine at the University of California David Geffen School of Medicine in Los Angeles. Those crummy feelings may be even more extreme if you're used to eating carb-heavy meals filled with bread and pasta. Cue the temptation to quit! A small study found that people who followed the paleo diet lost just over five pounds after three weeks. They also saw a 0.5-centimeter decrease in their waist circumference as well as improvements to their systolic blood pressure. (1) Systolic blood pressure refers to the pressure in your blood vessels when your heart is beating. Other research found that switching to a paleo diet led to short-term improvements in five components of metabolic syndrome (a risk factor for cardiovascular disease): waist circumference, triglyceride levels, blood pressure, HDL cholesterol, and fasting blood sugar.

*The Positive Long-Term Effects You May See From the Paleo Diet*
If you have weight to lose, you may or may not be able to keep weight off in the long term on the paleo diet. One study examined the effects of the diet on postmenopausal women with obesity after 6, 12, 18, and 24 months. The paleo group had lost significantly more weight compared with the control group (which followed a low-fat, high-carb diet) at the 6-month mark, but those results didn't carry over after 24 months. At the end of the two-year study, however, the participants who went paleo lost more fat and

saw greater improvement to abdominal obesity and triglyceride levels.

*The Possible Long-Term Disadvantages of the Paleo Diet*
One of the catches of this approach is you've got to stick to a paleo menu to see improvements. That seems obvious, but many people find it difficult to stay on track because the approach is restrictive and is not always conducive to traveling or eating out. Some experts say it's not an effective strategy for sustained weight loss for that reason. "Cutting out whole food groups, which is what the paleo diet does, results in a very restrictive diet, which is difficult to adhere to long term," Dolinski says. "The key to good nutrition is moderation, variety, and balance, and the paleo diet lacks variety and balance." Another barrier is that the diet can be expensive. Research suggests it can be 10 percent more costly than a diet with similar nutritional value. (7)

## Are You at Risk for Vitamin D Deficiency?

By cutting out entire food groups on the paleo diet, you may also miss out on key nutrients. Take dairy products like cheese, yogurt, and milk, for example. These can be great sources of calcium and vitamin D, both of which are critical to bone health, Dolinski says. One study found that people who followed a paleo diet had just 50 percent of the recommended dietary intake of calcium. (1) That's why nutrient deficiencies are one health risk of the paleo diet. Paleo dieters need to be careful about the types of meat they use to fill their plate. Red meat is high in saturated fat, which can raise blood cholesterol levels and increase the risk of heart disease and stroke. (8) Red meat should be consumed only in moderation, with no more than 13 grams of saturated fat per day if you're following a 2,000-calorie-per-day diet. (8) (If you're eating fewer calories, your saturated fat intake should be less.) That limit is easy to hit — a 3-ounce steak and a tablespoon of butter will put you over. Eating too much red meat can also be harmful to the kidneys, which play a role in metabolizing protein. One study found that replacing one serving of red meat with another type of protein — like chicken or seafood — can reduce the risk of end-stage kidney disease by 62 percent.

Even a 14-hour intermittent fasting window resulted in improved mood, sleep, and reduced hunger for nearly 40,000 people in a real-life trial.

Can the Paleo Diet Help Prevent Heart Disease?

When you think of ways to fight heart disease, adopting the so-called caveman diet might not immediately jump to mind as a tried-and-true option. But given that heart disease is the No. 1 killer in the United States — almost 700,000 Americans die from it every year — the search for solutions to improve heart health and prevent future heart events is understandably a concern for many. Over the past decade, researchers have explored whether the paleo diet — a restrictive approach based on the eating habits of our hunter-gatherer ancestors — can benefit people's heart health. So far, it's a mixed bag: Some findings are encouraging, while some members of the medical community remain skeptical about this diet plan.

Is the Paleo Diet Good for the Heart?

"Overall, the effect of the paleo diet on heart disease risk really depends on how you choose to follow it," says Kelly Kennedy, RD, a nutritionist for Everyday Health. Unlike other plans, the paleo diet doesn't recommend portion sizes by food group, nor does it incorporate exercise — which is known to be good for overall health and preventing heart disease. But following a paleo diet food list does require a focus on certain foods and the elimination of others. For instance, on the paleo diet, you're encouraged to eat lots of fruits, veggies, fats, and proteins, while processed foods like chips, cookies and candy, as well as legumes (beans), most dairy, and grains are off-limits.

## Tips for Eating Right to Prevent Heart Disease

This approach has pros and cons, Kennedy says. "My main concern overall would be the fact that major sources of fiber, vitamins, and minerals are being eliminated by not including whole grains, soy, and dairy," Kennedy explains. "However, if someone compensates and follows the paleo diet by having lots of fruits, vegetables, and lean protein sources such as skinless poultry and fish, they should be able to mostly compensate for these losses."

What Are the Benefits and Risks of the Paleo Diet?

There certainly has been a disconnect between some paleo enthusiasts and the medical community. For instance, while paleo recommends the elimination of whole grains, the American Heart Association states that whole grains can actually lower cholesterol and the risk of stroke, type 2 diabetes, and obesity. That being said, there are some encouraging signs out there. While some people may try the diet because they want to lose weight, when followed correctly, some studies suggest it could benefit your ticker. In fact, a systematic review from 2019 that looked at a wide range of relevant studies cited a number of potential heart health benefits, which were linked to the diet's cardio-friendly effects on areas like weight loss, body fat, and blood pressure. But the study noted that more research was needed to definitively establish a paleo-cardio connection.

The Diabetes Connection: Can Paleo Help?

One major risk factor for heart disease is type 2 diabetes. People who have type 2 diabetes can often develop hypertension, high cholesterol, and obesity — all major contributors to heart disease. Some research points to the potential of the paleo diet to help people with type 2 diabetes, but the overall body of evidence is mixed. A meta-analysis from 2020 of relevant research concluded that the paleo diet did not significantly affect diabetes or metabolic system any more than other diets perceived as "healthy." The researchers suggested that more studies with long-term follow-ups were needed to establish the true impact of the paleo diet on diabetes.

Using Paleo for Better Heart Health: Things to Keep in Mind

Kennedy urges people who are considering adopting paleo to realize that this diet allows for some foods that many experts do not consider heart healthy. She says that red meat and some of the saturated-fat-laden foods — such as ghee, coconut oil, and butter — may pose heart-health risks. "If someone eats those foods on a regular basis, their heart health will certainly suffer," she warns.

Red meat is one of the elements of paleo that causes experts, including Kennedy, to question whether it's good for heart health. Indeed, there's a growing body of literature that suggests eating too much red meat can harm the organ. (8) That doesn't mean you can't eat any red meat — just enjoy it in moderation. The American Heart Association (AHA) recommends choosing lean cuts when possible and opting for poultry and fish without skin — and prepared without saturated and trans fats — to protect your heart. If you need to lower your cholesterol, aim to reduce your saturated fat intake to a max of 5 to 6 percent of your total calories, or 13 g if you're consuming 2,000 calories per day.

Tips for Eating Right to Prevent Heart Disease

Kennedy also says it's important to remember that a heart-healthy diet is one that is low in sodium, and that while paleo may be naturally lower in sodium with the elimination of processed foods, paleo diets rarely come with "any recommended sodium restrictions." The most recent U.S. Department of Agriculture's Dietary Guidelines for Americans recommend that you consume no more than

2,300 milligrams (mg) of sodium per day. "In addition, when cutting out foods, such as legumes and whole grains, which are rich sources of fiber and some of the best cholesterol-lowering foods, it's not a good combination," she adds. Not only can removing whole food groups lead to nutrient deficiencies down the line, but if you're managing a condition such as type 2 diabetes — which can be better controlled with fiber — or have another underlying health issue, the paleo diet may have more cons than pros. Be sure to talk to your doctor before trying the paleo diet, especially if you have an underlying health condition.

# CONCLUSION

The paleo diet has been linked to weight loss and improvements to blood pressure and lipid profiles. But most research has been small in scope and conducted over a short period, so it's too soon to say conclusively what long-term effects you can expect after following the diet for years.